The
TRULY
NOURISHED
Detox & Plan for Life

A Healthier, Happier Version of YOU!

Hali Jafari is a Health and Lifestyle coach based in Bristol, UK. She has successfully lost 11 stone and kept it off for 2 years. During this time, she has helped many others reach their weight loss goals by introducing a plan she developed herself for her own weight loss journey.

In 2015 Hali won chef of the day on the cookery TV series The Box, presented by TV Chef James Martin. Her love of Middle Eastern food shows through in many of her recipes.

Hali has a passion for helping women become healthier and happier in their own skin, helping them gain confidence and live a fulfilling life by offering personal coaching sessions. You can find out more on her website:

www.trulynourished.co.uk

Table of Contents

Welcome   4
Introduction   6
What's the point?   8
Set your goals   9

The Detox   11
How do you measure?   12
Key points to remember   14
Detoxing food list   16
Keep note   20
Recipes for success   35
Breakfast   35
Lunch   40
Side dishes   46
Main meals   50

A Plan for Life   57
Life is for life   58
Points to remember forever   59
Foods to eat forever   61
Nourishing foods   64
Tracking   72
A change for life   73
Recipes for continuous success   74
Breakfast   75
Lunches and main meals   80
Side dishes   92
Desserts   97

Thank You   105
Notes   107

Welcome

Firstly, I'd like to personally thank you for being here and I'm truly honoured that you have given me the opportunity to show you a different, more holistic approach to weight loss, to build a positive relationship with food, and more importantly yourself!

I have struggled with my own weight and self-esteem issues since I was a child. I have tried every diet out there! In fact, I could probably tell you the calories, fat units, points and syn values of every food you could ever dream of consuming. I dieted, unsuccessfully, for over 20 years and each time a failed diet ended I would return to my previous weight, plus some added extra weight. Gradually I became bigger and bigger and by January 2013 and 3 children later I had reached my heaviest weight of 22 stone and a dress size 24/26.

I was morbidly obese, with a BMI of 47, and deeply unhappy. After many discussions with my family and months of debating if it was my last resort I decided to undergo weight loss surgery in August 2013 and had a gastric sleeve performed to help me with my battle of losing 11 stone in weight. My surgeon, Professor Ammori of the Manchester Spire Hospital, removed a portion of my overstretched stomach that would be a permanent tool to aid my weight loss. Whilst I don't think surgery is the answer to everyone's weight loss struggle, for me it was the tool I needed to help me begin losing my excess weight.

It took me only 8 months to lose 7 stone and it seemed so easy, my stomach was smaller and I could only eat 6 teaspoons of food at any one time, but then I hit a major plateau, my portion sizes were bigger and my weight stayed the same for over a month. I became frustrated and confused as to why the weight loss had slowed down so dramatically, but through determination and persistence I began to lose weight again after I retrained as a weight loss consultant and food psychology coach. I learned key factors about how the body uses certain foods for energy and how to lose weight more effectively by consuming foods that are good for the body, and achieve lasting results.

Teaming this knowledge with my flair for cooking delicious meals, I began to change my whole approach to my weight loss and realised that whilst smaller portions will always achieve weight loss there is more to losing weight successfully and keeping it off and that includes eating the right foods. While changing your mind-set at the same time.

During the 14 Day Detox Program you will be eliminating some of the most common foods attributed to weight gain, addiction, skin conditions and the general sluggishness of the digestive system.

This short term program will kick start your body into fat burning and flush toxins from the body ready for you to continue a healthy way of eating as you then move onto the Plan for Life. On the Plan for Life you will learn how to continue your weight loss in the long term; at this stage you will introduce some foods back into your diet to help make this a permanent lifestyle change that is easy, and enjoyable, to maintain.

I wish you all the best in your journey of self-confidence to help you reach a healthier, happier Truly Nourished you!

Hali x

P.S Please check with your doctor before embarking on any weight loss plan.

Introduction

The Truly Nourished Detox and Plan for Life has been designed to guide you through 6 weeks to a happier, healthier version of you.

Before you continue reading I would like you to do just one thing....

Forget everything you have ever been taught about dieting and weight loss. Have faith that you can change old habits and be successful in continuing to stay healthy and happy with the adaptations and changes you will make for the rest of your life.

The 14 Day Detox Program is where it all begins, it's where you will remove foods and chemicals from your diet than can typically leave you feeling ill, sluggish, tired and depressed. The 14 Day Detox Program will also encourage your body to burn fat and function better, as you will be consuming a large dose of vitamins, minerals and high energy foods that will satisfy your hunger and leave you feeling fantastic. There will be a few tough days to contend with as your body detoxifies and chemicals are eliminated, but this will only last a few days so please do not give up, it's all part of the process and will allow your body to function much better and boost your metabolism before you begin the Plan for Life on day 15.

The Plan for Life is a weight loss and maintenance stage, you are encouraged to stay on the Plan for Life for LIFE!

Your body will naturally reach its healthy weight if you continue on the Plan for Life. However we are all human and sometimes we want to enjoy special occasions such as a holiday or the festive season, which is why you can revert to the 14 Day Detox when it's needed, but please bear in mind you should leave around 12 weeks before detoxing again and only at a maximum of 4 times during the year.

The plan is very easy, it's all based on 'real' foods that are accessible to most of us through local grocers, health food shops and even supermarkets. I would suggest before you start either the 14 Day Detox Plan or the Plan for Life that you read the detoxing food lists and familiarise yourself with the foods you will be consuming, you may find you already have most of these food items in your kitchen anyway, be adventurous and try other foods that may not be familiar to you.

Shop in advance and ensure you are fully ready to get going before you start.

What's the point?

What's the point in embarking on a healthy eating program? Why are you doing this?
These are questions you must have clear answers for, without a goal there is no point in starting any new journey, plan, detox or program. Think carefully about what you want to achieve from this 14 Day Detox Program, and what your longer term goals are when you move onto the Plan for Life. Do you want to change your attitude to certain foods? Do you want more energy and a clearer mind? Or healthier skin? Do you wish to finally remove all negative association with diets and food? Would you like to reclaim your health and happiness?

Whatever your goals are, be specific and have something to aim for. Achieving something feels even better when you have determination for what's important to YOU! You may have short term and longer term goals that you wish to achieve, The 14 Day Detox Program encourages you to make short term goals, but have a think about your long term goals too where your health is concerned, and make some notes as you follow on through the program. Seeing your goals in black and white makes them more real and attainable.

Remember to focus on what you want, not what you don't want - for example instead of saying "I want to lose x amount of weight". Tell yourself "I want to reach a healthy size xx". Keeping your goals positive and focusing on what you want to have instead of not have will trick the brain into staying positive throughout your journey.

Believe you can and you are halfway there!

Set Your Goals

My short term goals:

1.

2.

3.

4.

5.

My long term goals:

1.

2.

3.

4.

5.

THE DETOX

How do you measure?

Please only measure and weigh yourself once on day 1 of the detox and the day after the last day of the detox.
Measuring and weighing yourself more than once a week will give you a false indication of how you are doing.
Weight loss is not always apparent until at least the first week is over and our bodies can either gain or lose up to 6lb in 24hrs!

Many things can affect your measurements and weight in any one day, these include the time of day you weigh, water retention, hormonal fluctuations, the weight of your clothes and also the size of the last meal consumed before weighing. Personally, I prefer to weigh once a month, in the morning and with no clothes to get a true picture of my weight.

For this 14 Day Detox I suggest taking your measurements as well as noting your weight on day 1 and day 15 (day after detox) to get a true reading of your results. May I also suggest you use a good set of digital weighing scales or, better still use the ones in your gym or chemist where you pay and get a full reading, these scales are calibrated regularly and there's no discrepancies with regards to uneven floors etc.

Don't let the scales rule your life!

Day 1

Weight ....ST.............LBS

Bust ....CM

Waist ....CM

Hips ....CM

Bottom ....CM

Thigh ....CM

Day 15

Weight ....ST.............LBS

Bust ....CM

Waist ....CM

Hips ....CM

Bottom ....CM

Thigh ....CM

Key Points to Remember

- This is a 14 DAY DETOX; it is not designed for you to continue for more than this period of time.

- It is only 14 days though so keep at it!

- It's not easy, but anything worth having never is.

- Listen to your body and only eat when you are hungry.

- Stop when you are full.

- Your last meal of the day should be consumed no later than 8pm.

- Eat at the table where possible with no other distractions.

- Savour each mouthful and do not rush your meal.

- Aim to take around 20 minutes to eat your meal, if you are quicker than this you are eating too fast, if you are slower than this you should stop at 20 minutes anyway as you have probably eaten enough.

- Use a side plate that looks full rather than a huge dinner plate that looks half empty.

- Don't snack between meals.

- Eat a variety from the food list, this will ensure you get a range of vitamins and minerals and prevent you from getting bored.

- Look at your food as fuel rather that satisfying cravings.

- Take a drink of water if you feel hungry between your meals, you are probably thirsty rather than hungry.

- Drink 30 minutes either side of your meal rather than with your meal. Drinking fluids when eating will encourage bloating and over stretching of the stomach.

- Remember to love yourself as you are, with the intention of creating a healthier, happier version of you.

Detoxing Food List

Each day choose 3 items from this list:
Blueberries (1 Handful)
Blackcurrants (1 Handful)
Blackberries (1 Handful)
Cranberries (1 Handful)
Raspberries (1 Handful)
Redcurrants (1 Handful)
Strawberries (1 Handful)
Gooseberries (1 Handful)
Grapefruit (1/2 a fruit)
Pomelo (1/4 of a fruit)
Melon (2 slices)
Mango (1/4 of a large fruit or ½ of a small fruit)
Apple (1 Fruit)
Pear (1 Fruit)
Kiwi (1 Fruit)

Each day choose 6-8 items from this list:
Asparagus (4 Stems)
Aubergine (1/2 a Vegetable)
Baby Corn (4 Vegetables)
Beetroot (1 Vegetable)
Broccoli (4 Florets)
Cabbage (2 Handfuls)
Cauliflower (4 Florets)
Celery (2 Whole Sticks)
Courgette (1/2 a Vegetable)
Cucumber (10cm Chunk approx.)
French Beans (10 Beans)
Fine Green Beans (10 Beans)
Kale (2 Handfuls)
Leeks (1Vegetable)
Lettuce (2 Handfuls)
Mangetout (10 Vegetables)
Mushrooms (5 Vegetables)
Peppers (1 Vegetable)
Radish (5 Vegetables)

Spinach (2 Handfuls)
Spring Greens (2 Handfuls)
Sugar Snap Peas (10 Vegetables)
Swede (4 tablespoons mashed)
Tomatoes (1 Fruit or 6 Cherry Tomatoes)
Turnip (1 Vegetable)
Vine Leaves (6 Leaves)
Watercress (2 Handfuls)

Each day choose 2 items from this list:
Sweet Potato (1 Vegetable)
Butternut Squash (1/4 Vegetable)
Carrots (1 Vegetable)
Parsnip (1 Vegetable)
Garden Peas (4 tablespoons)
Sweetcorn (4 Tablespoons)
Lentils (4 Tablespoons)
Butter Beans (4 Tablespoons)
Broad Beans (4 Tablespoons)
Chick Peas (4 Tablespoons)
Borlotti Beans (4 Tablespoons)
Pinto Beans (4 Tablespoons)
Black Beans (4 Tablespoons)
Red Kidney Beans (4 Tablespoons)
Black Eyed Beans (4 Tablespoons)
Aduki Beans (4 Tablespoons)
Split Peas (4 Tablespoons)
Wholegrain / Brown Rice (4 Tablespoons)
Spelt (4 Tablespoons)
Quinoa (4 Tablespoons)
Gluten Free Porridge Oats (25g)

Each day choose 3 items from this list:
Eggs (2 Eggs)
Tofu (size of the palm of your hand)
Chicken, skin Removed (size of the palm of your hand)
Turkey, skin Removed (size of the palm of your hand)
All Fish / Seafood
Avocado (1/2 a Fruit)
Nuts OR Seeds (1 Handful)
Vegan Protein Powder (1 Serving)

Each day choose 2 items from this list:
Cold Pressed Olive oil/ Avocado Oil (10ml)
Pure Coconut (Oil 2tsp)
Tahini Paste or Nut Butters (2tsp must be sugar free)
Homemade Hummus (2tbsp)

Each day choose 1 item from this list:
Manuka Honey (2tsp)
Whole Dates (maximum of 2)
Pure Maple Syrup (2tsp)

Each day choose freely from the following items in this list:
2 Litres of bottled or filtered water every day
Maximum of 1 Cup of Coconut Water per day
250ml of Dairy Free 'Milk' (i.e. Soya, Unsweetened Almond, Hazelnut or Coconut milk)
All Herbal and Fruit Teas (maximum of 3 per day)
Onions
Garlic
Lemons
Limes
All Herbs and Spices fresh or dried
Apple Cider Vinegar
Balsamic Vinegar
Himalayan Pink Salt
Black Pepper
Nutritional Yeast Flakes
Tomato Puree
Stevia Sugar Substitute

Please Note: For the whole 14 days you must NOT consume any Alcohol, Sugar or Dairy produce, this includes the following foods: All Artificial Sweeteners, Table Sugar, Brown Sugar, Regular Honey, Dried or Cooked or Tinned Fruits, Wine, Spirits, Beer, Butter, Cheeses, Yogurt, Cream, Tea, Coffee, Bread, Cakes, Crisps, Snacks, Chocolates, Ready meals, Tinned convenience foods (Only exception here is tinned pulses which should be drained and rinsed). Also, avoid takeaways and restaurants that cannot prepare your foods in the way acceptable on the plan.

Keep Note

Keep a journal for the 14 days; use a notebook or use the pages in the book to write in to jot down everything that passes your lips. You have 14 days to write down what you've eaten and any drinks you've consumed but do write it down straight away, all too often we can forget what we've eaten and munch on things mindlessly throughout the day, so noting everything as it happens will make you eat more consciously. Use your journal wisely and keep note of your feelings every day. How are you feeling? Excited? Happy? Tired? Headache? Whatever the feelings keep track, by the end of the 14 Days you will find all those feelings should be more on a positive note rather than negative.
Try to remember your goals every day to keep you on the right track.

Track the following every day:

FOOD ...

WATER INTAKE ...

HOURS OF SLEEP ...

NEGATIVE FEELINGS ...

POSITIVE FEELINGS ...

Day 1

FOOD

WATER INTAKE

HOURS OF SLEEP

NEGATIVE FEELINGS

POSITIVE FEELINGS

Day 2

FOOD

WATER INTAKE

HOURS OF SLEEP

NEGATIVE FEELINGS

POSITIVE FEELINGS

Day 3

FOOD

WATER INTAKE

HOURS OF SLEEP

NEGATIVE FEELINGS

POSITIVE FEELINGS

Day 4

FOOD

WATER INTAKE

HOURS OF SLEEP

NEGATIVE FEELINGS

POSITIVE FEELINGS

Day 5

FOOD

WATER INTAKE

HOURS OF SLEEP

NEGATIVE FEELINGS

POSITIVE FEELINGS

Day 6

FOOD

WATER INTAKE

HOURS OF SLEEP

NEGATIVE FEELINGS

POSITIVE FEELINGS

Day 7

FOOD

WATER INTAKE

HOURS OF SLEEP

NEGATIVE FEELINGS

POSITIVE FEELINGS

Day 8

FOOD

WATER INTAKE

HOURS OF SLEEP

NEGATIVE FEELINGS

POSITIVE FEELINGS

Day 9

FOOD

WATER INTAKE

HOURS OF SLEEP

NEGATIVE FEELINGS

POSITIVE FEELINGS

Day 10

FOOD

WATER INTAKE

HOURS OF SLEEP

NEGATIVE FEELINGS

POSITIVE FEELINGS

Day 11

FOOD

WATER INTAKE

HOURS OF SLEEP

NEGATIVE FEELINGS

POSITIVE FEELINGS

Day 12

FOOD

WATER INTAKE

HOURS OF SLEEP

NEGATIVE FEELINGS

POSITIVE FEELINGS

Day 13

FOOD

WATER INTAKE

HOURS OF SLEEP

NEGATIVE FEELINGS

POSITIVE FEELINGS

Day 14

FOOD

WATER INTAKE

HOURS OF SLEEP

NEGATIVE FEELINGS

POSITIVE FEELINGS

Recipes for Success

Here are some recipe ideas for you to try during the 14 Day Detox, I hope you enjoy them but that equally you get adventurous yourself in the kitchen and come up with your own recipes too. Also, look at ways you can adapt your usual favourite recipes using foods from the list provided.

Breakfast

Remember, it is the most important meal of the day, please do not skip breakfast! Your body works it's hardest to burn fat during the first half of the day and to boost this you should ideally begin the day with a hot water and lemon drink, which aids the body in flushing toxins that have built up during the night, and kick starts the metabolism ready for the day. After drinking your hot water and lemon make sure you eat a full breakfast, this could be porridge, a smoothie or fruit and nuts if you are short on time, but whatever you choose make sure it's consumed within an hour of waking to boost that metabolism.

Breakfast Super Smoothie
(Serves one)

Use a blender to combine the following ingredients and drink within 20 minutes before the vitamins begin to deplete! You could make up enough for a few days and freeze in batches ready to defrost in the mornings to save time.

Ingredients
1 Handful of Blueberries or strawberries
2 Sticks of Celery
2 Handfuls of Spinach
½ an Avocado
1 Cup of chilled Coconut Water
Squeeze of Lime
2 tsp of Manuka Honey

Egg and Soldiers
(Serves one)

Boil 2 organic eggs, aim to get the yolk runny for dipping! Use a combination of raw or lightly steamed asparagus, carrot and celery and cucumber sticks from your lists to use as your soldiers, plus 1 apple or pear (you don't have to use this to dip in your egg!)

Raspberry and Coconut Crumble
(Serves one)

Place a large handful of raspberries in a small baking dish and set aside, pre heat oven to 180 degrees. In a bowl, mix together 25g gluten free oats and 2 tsp melted pure coconut oil, 2 tsp Manuka honey and a small handful of desiccated coconut and flax seeds, spoon the mixture on to the raspberries and bake for 15 minutes. Enjoy hot or cold, this is one of my favourite breakfast recipes.

Banana and Date Bars
(Makes 16 portions)

Ingredients
200g Gluten free oats
100g Medjool dates
100g milled flax seed
100g chopped walnuts
100g melted coconut oil
1tsp ground cinnamon
3 mashed over ripe bananas
6tbsp honey
Method
Pre heat oven to 160 fan assisted. In a large mixing bowl, stir the oats, flax seeds, walnuts and cinnamon together. Melt the coconut oil together with the honey over a low heat, stirring continuously until melted, add the mashed bananas to the dry ingredients and mix well, pour the honey and oil mixture into the ingredients and combine well. Line a shallow brownie tray with baking paper, spoon mixture into lined tray and using the back of a metal soon evenly distribute the mixture and pat down to ensure mixture is compact and covered all over the tray, Bake at 160 fan assist for 20 minutes. Allow to cool in tray before cutting into equal bar portions. These bars are not crunchy; they are more a chewy texture so do not overcook.

Raspberry and Coconut Smoothie
(Serves one)

Ingredients
200ml Fresh coconut milk
100g Fresh raspberries
1tbsp milled flax seed 1/2 tsp ground cinnamon
Method
In a high-powered blender, add all ingredients and whizz on high speed for a couple of minutes to form a smooth a creamy consistency. Add ice if you prefer a cold and refreshing smoothie!

Oats and Blueberries
(Serves one)

Ingredients
25g Gluten free oats
100ml Dairy free milk (Almond or Coconut milk work well)
1 Handful of fresh blueberries
1/2 tsp ground cinnamon (Optional)
1tsp honey (Optional)
Method
Pour milk into saucepan and allow to warm up on a medium heat, before the milk begins to boil add oats and cook for approx. 5 minutes. If you require a little more milk for consistency, you can add more from your allowance keeping in mind your daily allowance of 250ml of dairy free milk. Pour cooked oats into serving bowl, sprinkle milled flax seeds and cinnamon over oats, add fresh blueberries (raspberries work well too as an alternative). Drizzle over honey and enjoy warm on a cold morning for a super boost of energy.

Lunch

Ahhh Lunch, that annoying meal in the middle of the day where a limp ham sandwich and a packet of crisps is deemed as a meal... please don't! Your body needs refuelling as the day goes on and you are busy rushing around at work, or with the children, or shopping until you drop! Stay focused and prepare in advance if you are out or at work for the day, a little forward planning will make or break your day on a detox. By this point of the day, you should have already consumed a litre of water so you shouldn't be starving and thirsty, so move on to your second meal of the day safe in the knowledge you are giving your body what it needs and deserves.

Balsamic Vegetables with Quinoa
(Serves four)

Nothing tastes as good as vegetables roasted in balsamic vinegar giving it a rich and sweet flavour. This salad is delicious warm but also tastes great as a cold lunch the next day.

Ingredients
1 red onion sliced
1 red pepper sliced
1 yellow pepper sliced
1 aubergine cut into chunks
Small punnet of baby plum tomatoes cut in half
3 or 4 garlic cloves sliced
150 ml balsamic vinegar
2tbsp olive oil
Himalayan pink salt and pepper to taste
1tbsp Manuka Honey
1 tin of cooked chick peas drained and rinsed
250g cooked Quinoa
1 handful of pine nuts

Method
Pre heat oven to 180 degrees fan assisted Place the red onion, peppers, aubergine, courgette, tomatoes and garlic cloves into a roasting pan, mix the balsamic vinegar and olive oil together before pouring over the vegetables, drizzle over the Manuka Honey and roast in a baking pan for around 40 minutes, checking occasionally. Once cooked remove from oven and allow to cool. In a large serving bowl add chickpeas, cooked quinoa, and toasted pine nuts (toast pine nuts by browning them in a hot dry frying pan) add the roasted vegetables to the Quinoa and chickpeas, add the toasted pine nuts, season with salt and pepper.

Shirazi Salad
(Serves four)

One of my favourite Persian go-to salads, which originates from the city of Shiraz.

Ingredients
Half a cucumber
2 tomatoes
Half a red onion or bunch of spring onions
2tbsp of chopped fresh dill
1 tsp olive oil
Juice of one fresh lime
Pinch of Himalayan Pink Salt
Method
Dice the cucumbers, tomatoes and onion into very small pieces, place into a salad bowl and add the dill, salt, lime juice and olive oil, mix together and serve with chicken, fish or enjoy on its own but make sure you add some nuts and seeds or avocado for essential fats and protein.

Roasted Aubergine Hummus
(Only 2tbsp recommended per serving on the detox)

The aubergine gives a creamy, silky texture to a classic hummus recipe, a great way to add more vegetables to your food without the kids even noticing!

Ingredients
1 Aubergine
1 red onion cut into wedges
2 cans of organic tinned chickpeas
2 cloves of garlic minced
5tsp tahini paste
80ml cooled boiled water
4tbsp freshly squeezed lemon juice
1/2tsp crushed Himalayan pink salt
100ml cold pressed olive oil, plus extra for drizzling, and to dress the hummus
Sprinkle of Paprika

Method
Preheat oven to 180 degrees fan assisted. Cut the aubergine in half and score the aubergine halves with a knife, drizzle with olive oil and add the onions, bake in foil for 30 minutes on medium heat or until fully cooked and you can scoop the middle out easily, leave the aubergine to cool. Meanwhile drain the chickpeas and rinse. Keep a few of the chickpeas aside for topping the hummus later, Place the rest of the chick peas, garlic, tahini paste, lemon juice and salt in a food processor and blitz, gradually add the olive oil and whizz again in processor, add the roasted aubergine and onions and whizz again! If your hummus is too stiff, you can add a little more cooled boiled water until soft enough for you. Place in dish, using back of a spoon create a dip in the middle and drizzle some olive oil over the hummus, sprinkle with paprika and add the chick peas that were kept aside for decoration. Serve with Crudités from your vegetable list.

Courgette, Spinach and Sweet Potato Burgers
(Serves two)

The whole family love these versatile veggie burgers, full of goodness and not a bit of processed meat in sight!

Ingredients
1 onion
2 courgettes
2 handfuls of fresh spinach
4 organic eggs
200g Cooked Sweet Potato
2tbs coconut oil
Method
Grate the onion and courgette and place in a sieve over a bowl, allow to drain for a few hours, pat with kitchen tissue and place in a large mixing bowl. Add the eggs and mix together with the courgette and onion. Mash the cooked sweet potato and chop the spinach, add all to mixture and season to taste. In a large frying pan warm the coconut oil on a medium heat, use an ice cream scoop to pick up mixture and gently place the 'burgers' in the hot oil to fry, cook on low-medium heat for around 10 - 15 minutes, gently turning over halfway through.

Roasted Turmeric Cauliflower and Kale

(Serves four)

Ingredients
1 Head of cauliflower, chopped and washed
1tbsp olive oil
1tbsp ground turmeric
1tsp Himalayan pink salt
16tbsp of Cooked spelt
50g Pumpkin seeds
4 Handfuls of fresh kale

Method
Pre heat oven to 180 degrees fan assisted. Place chopped cauliflower into a large pan, add enough boiled water to cover cauliflower and leave for 5 minutes to rest. Drain cauliflower in a colander, return to pan, pour the olive oil, turmeric and salt over cauliflower, place lid on pan, and give a good shake to ensure cauliflower is evenly covered in the oil and turmeric. Transfer cauliflower onto a baking tray and place on top shelf of oven. Roast for approx. 15 minutes and turn occasionally. On a serving plate, place a handful of kale per person, top with 4tbsp of cooked spelt and 4 cauliflower florets, top with seeds and serve.

Side Dishes

Some delicious recipe ideas to add to fish, chicken or tofu for a great meal.

Sweet Potato Wedges
(Serves one)

Ingredients
1 Sweet potato, chopped into wedges and washed
1tbsp olive oil
1tbsp ground turmeric
1tsp Himalayan pink salt
Method
Pre heat oven to 180 degrees fan assisted. Place chopped sweet potato onto a baking tray, drizzle in olive oil and sprinkle salt and turmeric over wedges. Place on top shelf of oven. Roast for approx. 30 minutes and turn occasionally. If after 30 minutes the wedges are not crisp enough, continue to cook until roasted to your liking.

Parsnip Crisps
(Serves one)

Ingredients
1 Parsnip
1tbsp olive oil
1tsp Himalayan pink salt

Method
Pre heat oven to 160 degrees fan assisted. Line a baking tray with some baking parchment. Using a vegetable peeler, shave the parsnip from root to tip. Place parsnip shavings onto a baking tray, drizzle in olive oil and sprinkle over the salt, using a spoon evenly coat the shavings by tossing and turning the parsnip shavings. Place on top shelf of oven. Roast for approximately 30 minutes. If after 30 minutes the parsnip is not crisp enough, continue to cook until nicely crisp. Transfer the crisps onto a cooling rack and allow to cool completely before serving.

Superslaw Warm Salad
(Serves four)

A delicious combination of fragrant, sweet and savoury flavours.

Ingredients
1 carrot grated
1 red onion sliced finely
½ head of green cabbage sliced finely
16tbsp cooked wholegrain rice
8 Medjool dates chopped
4 handfuls of chopped walnuts
1tbsp olive oil
1tbsp apple cider vinegar
1/2tsp of ground cinnamon
1tsp Himalayan pink salt

Method
Place all ingredients into a large frying pan and stir-fry for a few minutes before transferring into a large serving bowl, mix well and serve.

Cauliflower 'Rice' or 'Couscous'
(Serves four)

Great for when you need to bulk out a meal without resorting to carbs!

Ingredients
1 Whole cauliflower head
1tbsp coconut oil
1tsp Himalayan pink salt
Method
In a food processor blitz a head of cauliflower until it resembles a grain like texture. Lightly fry the 'rice' in the coconut oil and salt, you can add any herbs and spices to give more flavour if you wish. You can use the cauliflower 'rice' in place of rice or couscous in any recipe.

Main Meals

Here are a few Recipes for your main meals. Most people eat their biggest meal of the day in the evening, which is hard on our digestive system as it begins to slow down during the evening. Aim to eat no later than 7pm.

Superfood Salmon and Quinoa Salad
(Serves two)

This salad is a great way to boost your protein and fibre intake for the day; I usually make a big bowl and use up over a few days, great for packed lunches too.

Ingredients
120g cooked quinoa
1 small head of broccoli
8 cooked asparagus tips
2 handfuls of mixed seeds
2 grilled salmon fillets or fresh smoked salmon
5 radishes sliced Salad dressing
2tbsp apple cider vinegar
2tbsp cold pressed olive oil
A pinch of Himalayan pink salt and some black pepper to taste
Bunch of fresh chopped dill or coriander
Method
Mix the olive oil, vinegar, coriander, salt and pepper in a small bowl to make a dressing. Mix the remaining ingredients together in a large salad bowl and drizzle the salad dressing all over, enjoy!

Creamy Sweet Potato and Chickpea Curry
(Serves two)

I love this recipe, I make it really often as it is so easy to make and comforting to eat.

Ingredients
1tbsp coconut oil
1 large diced onion
2 garlic cloves minced
2 large sweet potatoes cut into 2cm cubes
1 can of chick peas in water drained and rinsed
160ml tinned coconut milk
1tbsp turmeric powder
1tsp of garammassala spice mix
1tsp of korma or curry powder
½ tsp of chilli powder
1tbs tomato purée
500ml water
Method
In a large saucepan fry onions and garlic together with turmeric, garamassala, curry powder and chilli powder for 5 minutes over medium heat. Add sweet potato and fry for further 10 minutes. Add chickpeas, water and tomato purée. Bring to boil then reduce to low medium heat, (do not place lid on saucepan), allow to simmer for around 20 minutes and if water has not reduced to half, turn up the heat a little. When water has reduced to half of original amount, add coconut milk and cook for further 10 minutes. Serve with brown rice, quinoa, cauliflower 'rice' or delicious on its own.

Chicken and Chips
(Seves 4)

Healthier version of a teatime classic that the whole family will enjoy.

Ingredients
8 chicken portions (drumsticks work well)
2 Limes
1 bunch of fresh chopped coriander
2tbsps of olive oil
Himalayan pink salt and black pepper to taste
2 large sweet potatoes peeled and cut into chunky size chips
2tbsp of olive oil
Himalayan pink salt
A sprinkle of paprika and turmeric
Method
Pre heat oven to 180 degrees. Line 2 baking trays with baking paper, in one of the prepared tins place some foil and place the chicken portions on the foil. Cut the 2 limes into wedges and place in between the chicken. Sprinkle over the coriander, salt and pepper and drizzle with the olive oil. Place some more foil on to prevent burning and place on the top shelf of oven and roast for around 20 minutes. Remove from oven and turn each piece over, cook for a further 10 minutes or until fully cooked. Remove the foil and roast for a further 10 minutes to brown. In the other tray place the chips on the baking paper, drizzle with olive oil, season with salt and sprinkle paprika and turmeric over the chips, mix well in the pan to coat the chips evenly, spread them out and roast for around 30 minutes. If you time it all well they should both be ready at the same time! Serve with large salad using vegetables from your list.

Roasted Butternut Squash and Pine Nut Salad
(Serves four)

Ingredients
2tsp Manuka honey
2tbsp coconut oil
2tsp chopped coriander
800g butternut squash, seeded and cut into wedges
2tsp apple cider vinegar
250g broccoli
400g tin red kidney beans, drained and rinsed
2 handfuls of fresh baby spinach
2tbsp lightly toasted pine nuts

Method
Preheat the oven to 180 degrees fan assisted. Line a large baking tray with baking paper. Combine half the honey with 1 tablespoon of melted coconut oil and the chopped coriander in a large bowl. Add the butternut squash and mix. Place on the lined tray and roast for 30–40 minutes or until golden, turning halfway through the cooking time. Meanwhile, combine the remaining honey and oil and the vinegar in a small bowl and set aside to use as a dressing.

Cook the broccoli in a saucepan of boiling water until just tender and drain, or steam lightly. Mix together the butternut squash, broccoli, red kidney beans, spinach and pine nuts in a large bowl. Add the salad dressing and gently mix to combine. Season to taste with sea salt and freshly ground black pepper.

Saffron Chicken with Tomatoes and Spinach
(Serves four)

The rich flavour from the saffron makes this dish fragrant and special, and gives a beautiful golden colour to the chicken.

Ingredients
1 onion diced
1 minced garlic clove
2tbs olive oil
1tsp of turmeric
1tsp of ground saffron
375g diced chicken breast
250g baby plum tomatoes
2 handfuls of sundried tomatoes
500ml of passata from jar
3 handfuls of fresh washed spinach
200ml water
Himalayan pink salt and black pepper to taste
Method
In a saucepan, fry the onions and garlic in the olive oil for 10 minutes until slightly browned. Add turmeric, saffron and chicken. Fry for a further 10 minutes on a medium heat. Add the baby plum tomatoes and the sun dried tomatoes and stir in the passata. Add the water and seasoning. Place lid on saucepan and simmer gently for 25 minutes, remove lid, add spinach and continue to simmer for a further 15 minutes or until sauce thickens. Serve with wholegrain basmati rice or quinoa.

Persian Chicken Skewers
(Serves four)

A healthier twist on a popular Persian dish usually served with boiled rice and salad.

Ingredients
4 diced chicken breast
1 grated red onion
1tsp of turmeric
1tsp of ground saffron
1tbsp of olive oil
1tsp of sea salt
6 wooden barbeque skewers
Method
Dip the ends of the skewers in a glass and pour enough water to cover the end of the skewers up to half way, put aside for now. In a large mixing bowl grate the onion, add the salt, turmeric, saffron, and mix. Pour in the olive oil and combine. Add the chicken to the sauce and leave to rest for 15 minutes. Pre heat oven to 180 degrees. Use some gloves to protect your hands from staining and place 3-4 pieces of chicken on to each skewer and rest on a baking dish or tray. Pour any remaining sauce over the skewered chicken and cook for around 30 minutes in the oven, turning the skewers around halfway through the cooking time. Check that the chicken is thoroughly cooked, remove from the oven, and serve with rice or salad.

No Deserts?

On the 14 Day Detox there is no room for desert or puddings as such I'm afraid, there are a few reasons for this;

It's an unnecessary habit to have a desert after a full meal, ask yourself if you really need something else to eat.

We are trying to adapt our taste buds a little throughout the detox in order for us not to give in to the sugar cravings, you will get deserts again after the detox, I promise!

If you really are a desert queen then please save a portion of your fruit allowance to have as a desert, try freezing berries as an alternative for sweets and different way to enjoy your fruit.

A PLAN FOR LIFE

Life is for LIFE!

Whether you have already completed the two weeks' detox, or you are just looking to make some healthier changes in respect to your body, your relationship with food and your self-esteem for life, then you are reading the plan that will help you in the healthiest way possible.

This plan aims to nourish your body from the inside out, you will feel lighter and healthier and this will show in your body, skin, your moods and your confidence. Most of us are fed so much conflicting advice as far as food and diet is concerned it's hard to know what to believe anymore. This plan takes us back to basics, to times where we didn't rely so heavily on convenience foods, eating out and takeaways, where we have no control of what chemicals and additives are going into our bodies. It also aims to help you break the traditional weight loss habits that over the years as a society we have believed to be the best way for us to lose weight i.e. counting calories and always eating low fat! Recent studies have proven time and time again that whilst portion control is important, counting calories and fat intake isn't as effective as we once thought, and in actual fact, we need good fats for health, it's more important to watch our sugar intake.

Therefore, if you are prepared to erase everything you have been taught regarding weight loss and are ready to take full control of your body then let us get started.

Here's to a Healthy, Happy you!

Hali x

Points to Remember Forever

- Listen to your body and only eat when you are hungry.

- Stop when you are full.

- Your last meal of the day should be consumed no later than 8pm.

- Eat at the table where possible with no other distractions.

- Savour each mouthful and do not rush your meal.

- Aim to take around 20 minutes to eat your meal, if you are quicker than this you are eating too fast, if you are slower than this you should stop at 20 minutes anyway as you have probably eaten enough.

- Use a side plate rather than a dinner plate that looks half-empty.

- Eat a variety of different foods to ensure you get a range of vitamins and minerals and prevent you from getting bored.

- Look at your food as fuel rather that satisfying cravings.

- Take a drink if you feel hungry between your meals, you are probably thirsty rather than hungry.

- Drink 30 minutes either side of your meal rather than with your meal. Drinking fluids when eating will encourage bloating and over stretching of the stomach.

- Remember to follow the plan at least 80% of the time allowing that 20% for treats on very important occasions and make the best choices you can every single day.

- Try to avoid alcohol where possible, alcohol is empty calories that contains very little nutritional value that will also make you crave salty, fatty foods.

- Drink as much water as you can manage, 2 litres is the recommended amount which equates to approximately 8 glasses per day.

- Don't weigh yourself every week!! People make this mistake repeatedly. It's important to understand that your body weight will fluctuate whether you are losing weight or not. Be kind to yourself, weigh once a month to get a true picture of your weight loss and use other ways to measure success, such as smaller clothes sizes and more self-esteem, and don't let the scales rule your life.

- Remember you are more than a number on the scales or a dress size, find other areas of yourself that you are happy with and focus on that.

- Self-esteem can be learnt! Look in the mirror every day and tell yourself you are beautiful, it's hard to do at first but you soon get used to it and then you start to believe it.

Foods to Eat Forever

Remember this is a Plan for Life. You now need to introduce some foods that were eliminated during the 14 Day Detox, these foods are good for you, and they are to be enjoyed every day and not to be thought of as a 'diet' food list. The foods listed below are foods to consume 80% of the time in order to stay healthy, leaving you room for 20% not so healthy foods, which can be enjoyed as part of life, after all we are human, we are here to live and enjoy social occasions where there may not be a healthy menu to choose from, or you may want to enjoy the odd glass of wine here and there.

Feel free to be in control of your own diet. You know what's good and what's not so good, so make healthy choices wherever and whenever you can so that when you want to have a coffee and a cake with friends you can do so without feeling guilty and enjoy yourself knowing that you haven't 'blown' your diet because this isn't a diet, this is a Plan for Life!

Fruits
All fruits, including dried, are great and should be consumed daily, a maximum portion or 3 per day is ideal to keep the sugar levels down. Do not use tinned fruits, which are usually in syrup or juice.

Vegetables
Aim for 6 to eight servings per day of ALL vegetables, keep your diet nice and varied to ensure a good variety of nutrients. Always remember that ½ of your plate should be filled with vegetables or salad at each meal. This will help fill you up as well as giving your body lots of vitamins, and fibre. Leafy greens should be included in at least two of your meals daily.

Protein
Protein is the secret to satiety. You should aim to consume a serving of protein at each meal to keep your energy levels up throughout the day and help keep you fuller for longer.
All sources of protein are advisable but avoid sources containing saturated fat such as hard cheese, fatty cuts of meat such as bacon, and any processed meats such as packaged cold meats, sausages, and any meats in tins or long life packaging.
Great sources are fee range and organic eggs, lean meats, poultry and pork, fish and seafood, quinoa, feta cheese, goat's cheese, all beans and pulses, avocados, nuts and seeds.

Complex Carbohydrates
This will be your trickiest food group to get right! Complex carbohydrates are the carbohydrates that have the least effect on sugar levels, always choose wholegrain and avoid bread, pasta and potatoes as much as you can. I like to use gluten free oats, spelt, pearl barley, freekah, wholegrain basmati rice, wholegrain couscous, bulgur wheat and buckwheat as my main sources of carbs. The odd white potato is not going to kill you though so do not deprive yourself of them just don't live on them at every meal.

Fats
There is so much information regarding fats that can be confusing for us but here are the best sources that are actually good for you and should be included in your meals daily. They will give you glowing skin, shiny hair and healthy nails: Nuts and seeds, including nut and seed butters, avocadoes and avocado oil, cold pressed olive oil, good quality pure coconut oil. If you are not going dairy free for life then butter from grass fed cows is ok. The only butters I have found to be grass fed are Kerry gold and Yeo Valley.

Sugar Substitutes

White table sugar has no nutrients and can cause havoc in the body by creating sugar rushes and cravings for high sugar and fatty processed foods, so avoid at all costs, find other alternatives to use in baking and drinks where necessary. Good substitutes that have a less damaging effect on the body include Manuka honey, natural date or fig syrups, Medjoul dates and dried fruits, pure maple syrup, Stevia and coconut palm sugar. Beware of agave nectar as it actually has a very high GI level, which will cause a sugar rush so use only occasionally. Finally avoid all chemical sugar substitutes such as sweeteners that contain aspartame, saccharin, acesulfame potassium, neotame and sucralose, as you can see by their names they sound pretty nasty and they are! So forget what you've learnt on diets that have encouraged you to use them. The other problem with using sweeteners is it doesn't train you to reduce your sweet tooth; you are replacing your sweet craving for chemicals instead.

A Note on Dairy...

After doing the 14 day detox you will be used to avoiding dairy and if you can continue without it that's great. Unsweetened soya milk in tea and coffee is great and coconut milk, rice milk or almond milk with oats in the morning or in a smoothie is a great alternative to cow's milk. There is lots of research to suggest cow's milk and produce is not easily digestible by the body and can contribute to many people suffering allergies and intolerance's, as well as bloating, eczema, acne, and inflammation of the joints. This is where you make up your own mind on the great dairy debate. Personally I avoid it in most cases as I find my skin clears up, migraines are less frequent, and as an arthritis sufferer, I find my joints ache much less without it. I prefer to use feta and goat's cheese in recipes and occasionally butter from grass fed cows. I find eating dairy very rarely okay for me, but some people do prefer to quit dairy from their diet entirely.

Nourishing Foods

'You are what you eat' as they say, so choose the best you can afford as far as good foods go. Buy organic if you can, or at least free range, fresh and colourful foods. After all who doesn't want to feel great every day?

The key to nourishing your body from inside out is to ensure you are eating from a wide range of vitamins and minerals and from all the food groups. If you have read the Truly Nourished 14 Day Detox Plan then you will already be familiar with some of the great foods that should be consumed regularly, but here is a list of the various nutrients you should be consuming and in which foods you can find them.

Vitamin A
Vitamin A should be avoided during pregnancy but for everyone else it's an essential vitamin that is particularly amazing for our skin as it helps the production of skin cells, aiding cell turnover, repair and renewal. It also defends our skin from UV damage and is an important immune booster.
You can find Vitamin A in the following foods:
• Sweet Potatoes
• Butternut Squash
• Pumpkin
• Carrots
• Kale
• Spinach
• Romaine Lettuce

Vitamin B1 (Thiamine)
Vitamin B1 is essential for energy production and helps support the nervous and digestive system.
You can find Vitamin B1 in the following foods:
• Sunflower seeds
• Nuts
• Peas
• Brussels Sprouts
• Lentils and Black Beans

Vitamin B2, B3, B5, B6 & B7
I have grouped these B vitamins together mainly because whilst they do some separate things they also have a lot in common as to being essential for healthy skin, hair and nails as well as aiding skin cell renewal and DNA repair.
You can find the above B Vitamins in the following foods:
• Spinach
• Salmon
• Sardines
• Asparagus
• Eggs
• Avocado
• Mushrooms
• Nuts
• Seeds

Vitamin B9 (Folate)
Vitamin B9 isn't talked about much but if you are pregnant it's essential for a healthy pregnancy as well as helping to repair cells.
You can find Vitamin B9 in the following foods:
• All leafy greens
• Asparagus
• Brussels Sprouts
• Lentils
• Chickpeas

Vitamin B12
Vitamin B12 is essential for energy, metabolism, brain and nerve function. This is an important one as deficiency in this vitamin can leave you lethargic, tired and suffering with 'brain fog'.
You can find Vitamin B12 in the following foods:
• Salmon
• Sardines
• Meat
• Eggs
• Shellfish

Vitamin C
Vitamin C is an important and powerful antioxidant; it's also essential for the formation of collagen and elastin in the skin which helps keep it firm and toned.
You can find Vitamin C in the following foods:
• Strawberries
• Pineapple
• Papaya
• Kiwi
• Red, yellow and orange Bell Peppers
• Kale
• Cabbage
• Brussels Sprouts

Vitamin D

Whilst vitamin D is difficult to get enough of from food alone, every little helps especially if you live in a cold climate where you may not see enough sun, which is the body's most effective way of making the vitamin. Lack of vitamin D can have many symptoms such as low mood, tiredness and lethargy and achy bones.

You can find Vitamin D in the following foods:
• Eggs
• Sardines
• Mushrooms
• Almond Milks fortified with additional Vitamin D

Vitamin E

Vitamin E is another skin saver, helping to protect against damage from free radicals and supporting the skin by helping to maintain moisture levels in the skin and scalp. A great anti-aging vitamin!

You can find Vitamin E in the following foods:
• Spinach
• Tomatoes
• Peaches
• Papaya
• Avocado
• Olive oil and olives
• Nuts &Seeds

Vitamin K

An important vitamin for healthy teeth, nails and strong bones, as well as being essential for healthy blood clotting, preventing varicose veins and reducing dark circles under the eyes.

You can find Vitamin K in the following foods:
• Asparagus
• Broccoli
• Brussels sprouts
• Spinach
• Kale
• Cauliflower
• Cucumber
• Red Cabbage
• Basil and Parsley

Co-Enzyme Q10
Co-Enzyme Q10 helps to keep cell membranes strong and provide them with energy. Co-Enzyme Q10 is great for defending against fatigue and heart conditions and helps to support a healthy metabolism.
You can find Co-Enzyme Q10 in the following foods:
• Sesame Seeds
• Walnuts

Calcium
Calcium is essential for healthy teeth, bones and nails, as well as calming the nervous system. We need Calcium to support cell renewal and wound repair in the body. The great news is you don't just have to drink cow's milk to get calcium, as you can find Calcium in the following foods:
• Spinach
• Peaches
• Papaya
• Avocado
• Olive oil and olives
• Nuts &Seeds

Copper
Copper is important for nervous function, great for healthy hair, skin and nails and helps to build bones and connective tissue.
You can find Copper in the following foods:
• Apricots
• Pineapple
• Goji Berries
• Cashew Nuts
• Coconut
• Pumpkin Seeds
• Tahini
• Lentils
• Leafy Greens

Iron

Iron is essential for the formation of red blood cells in the body and transporting oxygen in the blood. We need Iron for energy but it also helps to maintain healthy nails and shiny hair.

You can find Iron in the following foods:

- Kale,
- Spirulina
- Pumpkin seeds and Hemp seeds
- Walnuts
- Lentils and red meat
- Potatoes

Magnesium

One of the reasons we are said to crave chocolate is due to a deficiency in this mineral! Magnesium helps with PMS symptoms and helps to calm the nervous system and reduce stress and anxiety.

You can find Magnesium in the following foods:

- Quinoa
- Cashew Nuts
- Coconut
- Pumpkin Seeds
- Oatmeal
- Leafy Greens
- Courgettes

Manganese

Manganese helps to build strong boners and connective tissue; it also helps the body to heal wounds. Healthy hair and hair colour is also a bonus from this mineral.

You can find Manganese in the following foods:

- Spinach
- Potatoes
- Green Tea
- Cinnamon
- Oats
- Chickpeas
- Pecans
- Pineapple
- Figs

Omega Fatty Acids
Fatty Acids are essential for brain and eye health and helps to regulate our hormones and mood. It also contains anti-inflammatory nutrients and strengthens the skin barrier.
You can find Omega Fatty Acids in the following foods:
• Chia seeds and Hemp seeds
• Flax seeds (Linseeds)
• Salmon
• Trout
• Sardines
• Walnuts

Potassium
Important mineral for healthy circulation, muscle and nerve function in the body, great if you suffer with muscle cramps! Potassium also aids the PH balance in the body.
You can find Potassium in the following foods:
• Bananas
• Butternut Squash
• Chard
• Potatoes
• White Beans

Selenium
Helps to maintain elastin in the skin and protect against damage from free radicals.
You can find Selenium in the following foods:
• Coconut Water
• Brazil Nuts
• Oats

Zinc

Zinc is essential for healing of the skin and fight inflammation, particularly essential for those suffering with acne or eczema. It also helps to build collagen in the skin which strengthens the skin helping it to stay firm and toned.

You can find Zinc in the following foods:

• Quinoa
• Walnuts
• Tahini
• Pecans
• Chia seeds
• Pumpkin seeds
• Chickpeas
• Mushrooms
• Shellfish

Tracking

Remember the 14 Day Detox Program Daily Diary? Well I suggest for the next 28 days you do the same again. I know it's boring and time consuming which is why I suggest you find your own way of keeping note of your daily food intake either by writing it down in a separate little notebook, or use your phone, the notes section in your phone is great for this or you could download the many free food intake apps there are nowadays. I actually find the best way for me is to take pictures of my meals using my phone, of course this does mean that I have a phone full of food pictures but it does keep me on track and if I come up with a nice new recipe, it means I have a picture to go with it. Whatever way you decide to keep tracking your daily intake I strongly advise you to do it for the next 28 day at least, this is because you are still learning, you may forget something you've eaten and whilst we are no longer following the detox which is a little stricter, it does keep you focused until the foods and lifestyle choices you make become automatic and don't require as much thought.

Track the following every day:

FOOD …

WATER INTAKE …

HOURS OF SLEEP …

NEGATIVE FEELINGS …

POSITIVE FEELINGS …

A Change for Life

As with the detox, this plan requires some life changing decisions based on your food choices, so if you chose to treat this as a diet rather than a plan for life, you will give in at some point and return to your old eating habits. That is why I believe in the 80/20 rule (80% healthy eating for life and 20% room for special occasional treats) so you don't feel you are on a restrictive plan.

As you can see, there are no calories to count, but portion control is just as important as the foods you eat. There is no need to eat more than a side plates worth of food at any one sitting. Think of the size of your stomach and how you are over stretching it each time you over eat, this will cause your stomach to grow bigger and need more food to fill in order for you to feel satisfied. Also our bodies can only use so much food as fuel at any one time so if you eat a larger meal than is needed your body will store the rest of the energy from that meal as reserve energy, which if not burned off with exercise, will turn into body fat.

Talking of exercise, aim for 30 minutes of activity per day but chose something you enjoy. I've spent many years, and a lot of money on gym memberships that I have not made full use of but that's because I prefer a nice walk in the woods or a belly dancing class or exercising at home, but if you like the gym or group exercise then do it and enjoy it. We all need some me time every day and exercise is the perfect way to let off steam, relax or have fun as well as burning off some excess energy in the body.

Please note though that, whilst exercise is an important part of staying healthy, it will not allow you to eat a mars bar because you did an hour long run! Your diet will still determine around 70-80% of how effective your weight loss can be. So do the exercise in the knowledge you are gaining strength and releasing happy hormones that will keep you on track and still stick to the healthy eating to get the best results.

Your mind, body and soul will thank you for it.

Recipes for Continuous Success

Here are some recipe ideas for you to use on a daily basis, they can always be adapted if there is a certain ingredient you are not keen on in a recipe. Once again remember the importance of eating a variety of meals and ingredients to ensure you are getting all the nutrients your body needs and craves, as well as making healthy eating a bit more exciting than the same tuna salad every day!

Breakfast

Almond and Cranberry Bars
(Makes 16 bars)

Keep fresh in an airtight container for around 3 days, you can also freeze them if any leftover!

Ingredients
100g gluten free oats
180g ground almonds
150g dried cranberries
150g Honey
1tsp ground cinnamon
3tbsp walnut oil
For the topping
100g mixed seeds
1tbsp flaked almonds
1tbsp honey
Method
Preheat oven to 160 degrees (fan assisted) and line a shallow brownie tin with some baking parchment. Mix the oats, ground almonds, cranberries, cinnamon, honey and walnut oil; you should get a stiff mixture. Using the back of a metal spoon pat the mixture into the lined baking tin ensuring a level finish, sprinkle the seeds and flaked almonds over the mixture and drizzle the honey over the top. Bake for around 20 minutes Allow to cool completely before cutting into finger size bars, even better leave them for at least 6 hours before eating as they will set well.

Banana, Walnut & Honey Breakfast Bars
(Makes 16 bars)

These bars are not crunchy; they are more of a chewy texture so do not overcook.

Ingredients
200g gluten free oats
100g milled flax seed
100g chopped walnuts
100g melted coconut oil or butter
1tsp ground cinnamon
3 mashed over ripe bananas
6tbsp honey
Method
Preheat oven to 160 fan assisted. In a large mixing bowl, stir the oats, flax seeds, walnuts and cinnamon together. Melt the coconut oil (or butter) together with the honey over a low heat, stirring continuously until melted, add the mashed bananas to the dry ingredients and mix well. Pour the honey/ oil mixture into the ingredients and combine well. Line a shallow brownie tray with baking paper. Spoon mixture into lined tray and using the back of a metal soon evenly distribute the mixture and pat down to ensure mixture is compact and covers the entire tray. Bake at 160 degrees in a fan assisted oven for 20 minutes. Allow to cool in tray before cutting into finger size portions.

Coconut Couscous Mini Muffins
(Makes 24 mini muffins)

Ingredients
80g cooked giant wholegrain couscous
160ml coconut cream
2tbsp chia seeds
50g coconut flour
3tbsp desiccated coconut
3 handfuls fresh blueberries
2tbsp agave syrup
3tbsp mixed seeds of choice
Method
Preheat oven to 160 degrees fan assisted. Line a mini
cupcake/ muffin tray with mini cases. Mix all ingredients
together in a bowl saving some blueberries for decoration.
Use a small spoon to fill each case with mixture and top with a
blueberry. Bake for 30 minutes, remove from oven and allow
to cool before serving.

Rhubarb and Cherry Breakfast Crumble
(Serves four)

This breakfast crumble is so delicious, perfect on a cold winter's morning, I quite often make it all the night before and then just pop in the oven in the morning to save on time.

Ingredients
5 stems rhubarb chopped
100g frozen cherries
2tbsp honey
100g gluten free oats
30g linseeds
2tbsp mixed seeds
50g melted organic butter or coconut oil if dairy free
Method
Preheat oven to 150 degrees fan assist. Cook rhubarb and cherries with the honey and 1tbsp water for 10 minutes, pour into baking dish. Mix the oats, linseeds and seed mix and sprinkle over the rhubarb and cherry mixture. Melt the butter and drizzle all over. Cook for 25 minutes, enjoy hot or cold.

Coconut and Raspberry Breakfast Muffins
(Makes 24)

Yummy at breakfast or mid-afternoon for a boost of energy thanks to the slow energy releasing oats!

Ingredients
250ml unsweetened coconut or almond milk
200g gluten free oats
100g linseed/ chia seed mix
60g desiccated coconut
100g coconut palm sugar
100g coconut flour
200g honey
3 eggs
100g melted pure coconut oil
300g fresh raspberries
1tsp baking powder
Method
Preheat oven to 150 (fan assisted) and line a cupcake tray with 24 cases. In a mixing bowl add the coconut palm sugar, oats, linseed/ chia seeds, desiccated coconut, coconut flour and baking powder. In a jug whisk together the eggs and honey and add the milk, pour over dry ingredients and combine. Pour in melted coconut oil and mix well. Finally add the fresh raspberries and fold into the mixture. Using an ice cream scoop, spoon in a level scoop of mixture into baking cases and bake for 25/30 minutes, remove from oven and place onto a cooling rack to cool.

Lunches & Main Meals

Some great ideas for the main meals of the day, make sure you switch it up a bit, ensure you eat a variety of foods and listen to your body to see when you are really hungry and when you are full make sure you put down the knife and fork.

Balsamic Vegetables with Pine nuts and Feta
(Serves four)

Ingredients
1 red onion sliced
1 red pepper sliced
1 yellow pepper sliced
1 aubergine cut into chunks
Small punnet of baby plum tomatoes cut in half
3 or 4 garlic cloves sliced
150 ml balsamic vinegar
2tbsp olive oil
Salt and pepper
1tbsp coconut palm sugar
1 tin of cooked chick peas
250g mixed grains cooked
1 handful of pine nuts
40g feta
Method
Preheat oven to 180 degrees fan assisted. Place the red onion, peppers, aubergine, tomatoes and garlic cloves into a roasting pan. Mix the balsamic vinegar and olive oil together before pouring over the vegetables. Sprinkle over the coconut sugar, roast for around 40 minutes, checking occasionally. Once cooked, remove from oven and allow to cool.
In a large serving bowl add chick peas, cooked mixed grains (quinoa, barley, bulgur wheat), and toasted pine nuts (toast pine nuts by browning them in a hot dry frying pan) Add the roasted vegetables in to the grains and chick peas, add the toasted pine nuts, season with salt and pepper and add chunks of feta cheese.

Coconut and Lime Prawns with Soba Noodles and Avocado
(Serves four)

This is my 14 year olds favorite meal and it's so quick and easy to make.

Ingredients
1tbsp coconut oil
500g fresh king prawns
200g Soba Noodles
1tbsp coconut cream (comes in a firm block)
Juice of one fresh lime
2 yellow bell peppers sliced
1 ripe avocado
1tsp Himalayan pink salt
Method
Bring a large pan of water to boil and add soba noodles, turn down heat and allow to cook for 5/10 minutes, drain and set aside. In a large frying pan melt the coconut oil, add the prawns, lime juice and salt and fry until prawns are cooked. Add the soba noodles to the frying pan with the cooked prawns and add the creamed coconut. Stir until the creamed coconut has melted. Warm through for few minutes before adding the peppers and avocado. Mix well and serve in bowls.

Turkey Chili
(Serves four)

Perfect way to lighten up a traditional Chili Con Carne is to use turkey mince instead of red meat.

Ingredients
2 onions diced
2 garlic cloves minced
2tbsp olive oil
500g lean turkey mince or soya mince
300g red kidney beans soaked overnight or use 1 tin in water drained
1 aubergine diced
1 courgette diced
2tsp turmeric powder
2tsp Paprika
Chilli powder to taste
Salt and pepper to taste
1tsp stevia powder
4tbsp tomato puree
1 Carton or jar of passata (500ml)

Method
Fry the onion in the olive oil until it softens. Add the garlic, turmeric, paprika and chilli powder and continue to fry for a few minutes before adding the minced turkey. Fry all together until meat has lost its pinky colour. Add the diced aubergine and courgette and stir well, add the salt and cook for a further 5-10 minutes before adding the red kidney beans, tomato puree and Passat. Add the water and tsp of stevia and bring to a boil before allowing to simmer for approx. 30 minutes or until you have the desired consistency. Serve with Wholegrain Rice, cauliflower rice or quinoa.

Quick and Easy Tuna Salad
(Serves one)

Mix together 1 can of tuna in spring water, ½ a cupful of cooked sweetcorn, ½ an avocado and a large handful of baby leaf salad. For Salad Dressing: 1 tsp olive oil, salt and pepper, ¼ tsp mild mustard, 1tsp white wine vinegar mix all together for a delicious salad dressing.

Butternut Squash with Puy Lentils, Feta and Rocket
(Serves one)

Ingredients
60g of cooked puy lentils
100g of cooked butternut squash
Matchbox size of feta cheese crumbled
Large handful of fresh rocket leaves
Method
Mix all ingredients together for a quick and easy meal that's full of goodness! You could add a little balsamic vinegar as a dressing if you like and season with some Himalayan pink salt.

Feta, Fig and Avocado Salad
(Serves one)

In a bowl mix together ½ an avocado, 2 fresh figs chopped, a matchbox size of feta cheese crumbled, ½ a cupful of cooked mixed grains (barley, quinoa, and spelt are a good mix), 1 yellow pepper chopped, 1 tsp olive oil and top with 1tbsp of chopped walnuts. This salad doesn't really need a dressing due to the juicy figs but feel free to add some apple cider vinegar to add a little oomph to the salad!

Peanut Butter Tofu with Sesame Soba Noodles and Broccoli

(Serves four)

Ingredients
2tbsp of peanut butter
500g Tofu
200g Soba Noodles
1tbsp soy sauce
1tsp honey
2tbsp sesame seeds

Method
Place broccoli in a steamer for 15 minutes. Bring a large pan of water to boil and add soba noodles, turn down heat and allow to cook for 5/10 minutes, drain and set aside.
Place peanut butter in frying pan, cut up the tofu into chunks, place in frying pan with peanut butter. Turn hob on to medium heat and start to coat the tofu in peanut butter, continue to fry for 10 minutes until tofu cooked and browned. Remove from heat and place tofu pieces on plates, return the soba noodles in the frying pan used for tofu, turn on heat to medium, add sesame seeds, soy sauce and honey and warm through for few minutes. Broccoli should now be cooked and ready, add some soba noodles to the tofu on plates and add some broccoli, enjoy!

Hearty Bean & Barley Soup
(Serves four)

A really filling, delicious and warming, my most favourite soup ever!

Ingredients
1 onion diced
2 carrots sliced
2 handfuls of pearl barley rinsed
1 can of chick peas in water drained
1 can of red kidney beans in water drained
1 can of butter beans in water drained
4tbsp tomato puree
600ml water
Method
Place all ingredients in a large saucepan and bring to the boil, reduce heat and simmer until thoroughly cooked and the soup has thickened.

Veggie Frittata with Mozzarella & Avocado Salad
(Serves four)

Ingredients
6 large free range organic eggs
1tsp olive oil
4 mushrooms sliced
1 courgette sliced
10 cherry tomatoes sliced in half
Mixed green salad leaves
5 cherry tomatoes
½ avocado cubed
12 mini mozzarella pearls
Splash of balsamic vinegar for salad dressing

Method
In a bowl whisk all the eggs together, season with salt and pepper if you wish. Warm the olive oil in a large frying pan, place the mushrooms, courgette and cherry tomato halves in the frying pan and cook for 5 minutes until softened. Pour over whisked eggs and cook on a low heat, after 10 minutes place the frying pan under a hot grill to cook the top of the frittata. Remove from grill and cut into 8 wedges, serve with the mixed salad leaves, cherry tomatoes, avocado and mozzarella and add a splash of balsamic vinegar as a dressing.

Chickpea, Pistachio, Feta & Caramelised Red Onion Couscous
(Serves four)

Ingredients
250g cooked couscous
1 red onion
1tbsp olive oil
2tbsp balsamic vinegar
2tsp coconut palm sugar
1 can of chick peas in water drained
Handful of chopped pistachios
50g feta cheese crumbled

Method
In a large frying pan fry the onion in the olive oil on a low heat for 5 minutes, add the balsamic vinegar and turn up the heat to medium, cook for further 5 minutes or until vinegar has evaporated. Add the coconut palm sugar and cook for further 5 minutes until onions have caramelised stirring continuously. In a large bowl add the cooked couscous, chickpeas, pistachios and caramelised onion and stir well. Finally crumble the feta on top and serve. Add a green salad to this for extra goodness.

Spelt and Halloumi Stuffed Bell Peppers

A healthier adaptation of a traditional Persian family favourite.

Ingredients
4 bell peppers
1 small onion diced
1 garlic clove minced
1tbsp olive oil
1tsp turmeric
6tbsp cooked spelt
Handful of mixed herbs
1tsp cinnamon
2tbsp yellow split peas cooked
Juice of 1 lime
6tbsp water
2tsp tomato puree
6 sundried tomatoes chopped
4 slices of halloumi cheese
Method
In a large frying pan, warm the olive oil, add the onion, garlic and turmeric and fry until onions are soft. Add the cooked spelt, herbs, cinnamon, cooked yellow split peas, lime juice, water, tomato puree and chopped sun dried tomatoes and cook for a further 10 minutes. Slice the tops from the bell peppers and place in a baking dish that fits all 4 peppers comfortably so they are snug in the baking dish, stuff each pepper with equal amounts of the filling and top with a slice of halloumi cheese. Place the head of pepper back on top and secure with a cocktail stick. Bake in a pre-heated oven at 170 degrees fan assisted for around 40 minutes until peppers are cooked and soft.

Baby Potato, Kale and Egg Bake
(Serves four)

Ingredients
250g baby new potatoes, par boiled for 10 minutes
3tbsp olive oil
1tsp sea salt flakes
½ a red onion
2 handfuls of white cabbage
4 handfuls of fresh kale
6 eggs
Method
Preheat oven to 180 degrees fan assisted, in a large baking tray place all the par boiled baby potatoes on some baking parchment, sprinkle with salt and drizzle over 2tbsps of the olive oil, bake for around 30 minutes until roasted. Place the red onion, cabbage and kale into a large frying pan and pour over the remaining 1tbsp of olive oil, fry for 10 minutes until slightly softened. Take a large baking dish, something suitable for a family sized lasagne is great. Place the roasted baby potatoes on the bottom of the baking dish, top with the onion, cabbage and kale and finally crack open the eggs on the top. Bake for around 10 minutes and serve.

Mixed Vegetable and Turmeric Pilaf

(Serves four)
Another Persian favourite that's very tasty thanks to all the warm spices used to give flavor and colour.

Ingredients
250g cooked wholegrain basmati rice
1 onion diced
1 clove of garlic minced
1 large carrot diced
2 handfuls of trimmed green beans, cut into 1 inch lengths
1 medium potato diced
1tbsp olive oil
2tbsp tomato puree
300ml cold water
2 tsp turmeric powder
1 tsp cinnamon powder
½ tsp chili powder

Method
In a large frying pan, fry the onion, garlic, turmeric, cinnamon and chilli powder in the olive oil for 5 minutes. Add all the vegetables and fry for a further 10 minutes. Transfer to a large saucepan and add the tomato puree and water, bring to boil then reduce heat to simmer, continue to cook until most of the water evaporates and you are left with a very thick sauce. Add the rice to the vegetables and mix, cook for a further 5/10 minutes to ensure the rice is cooked through.

Wholegrain Rice & Lentil Salad

Literally the easiest salad to make ever!

Ingredients
4tbsp wholegrain rice
4tbsp of puy lentils
1 grated carrot
1 handful of chopped cucumber
1tbsp of raisins
1tbs sesame seeds
The juice of half a lemon
Method
Just mix together and enjoy!

Side Dishes

Rosemary and sea salt crushed potatoes
(Serves four)

Ingredients
4 large Maris piper potatoes
2tbsp olive oil
Pinch of sea salt flakes
Bunch of fresh rosemary
Method
Preheat oven to 180 degrees fan assisted. Bring a large pan of water to the boil. Wash the potatoes, leaving the skin on, Cut potatoes into quarters add to boiling water and par boil for 10 minutes, drain and place on kitchen towel and gently pat dry. In a large baking tray add 1tbsp of olive oil to the tray and place potatoes on tray, use a fork to gently crush the potatoes and pour the remaining tbsp. olive oil over the potatoes, sprinkle with sea salt and place rosemary over potatoes. Place baking tray in the oven and cook for around 40 minutes, turning the potatoes around halfway through cooking.

Sprouts and Chestnuts

I absolutely love chestnuts, and nothing tastes as good with them as Brussels sprouts lightly stir fried together in coconut oil, and a pinch of sea salt flakes. Tastes good with any meal!

Healthier Chips!
(Serves four)

Ingredients
4 large Maris piper potatoes
2tbsp olive oil
A pinch of sea salt flakes
Method
Preheat oven to 180 degrees fan assisted. Bring a large pan of water to the boil. Wash and peel the potatoes, Cut potatoes into equal sized chips, add to boiling water and par boil for 10 minutes, drain and place on kitchen towel and gently pat dry. Place the chips onto a large baking tray and pour over olive oil, sprinkle with sea salt and place in oven on top shelf and cook for around 40 minutes, turn the chips over around halfway through cooking.

Roasted Garlic Aubergines

(Serves four)

A perfect side dish that goes well with so many foods

Ingredients
2 large aubergines
1 bulb of garlic
1 red onion
2tbsp olive oil
Salt and pepper to taste

Method
Preheat oven to 160 degrees fan assisted. Cut the aubergines in half and score through and vertically down the middle of the vegetable and score a few horizontal lines across (as shown in photo). Line a baking tray with some foil. Slice some of the garlic cloves into slivers and place into the scored aubergines. Place the remaining garlic cloves on to the baking tray. Cut the red onion into wedges. Place the aubergine halves and red onion wedges onto foil and sprinkle with salt and pepper and drizzle with olive oil. Bake for around 40 minutes or until aubergine is soft and cooked well. Scoop out the flesh and enjoy with any meal.

Spicy Bean and Seed Mix
(Serves four)

A really tasty snack that will satisfy cravings for salty fatty snacks. Much tastier, healthier and filling.

Ingredients
1 can of chick peas
1 can of red kidney beans
1 can of pinto beans
2tbsp each of sunflower seeds, pumpkin seeds, pine nuts, linseeds and sesame seeds
1tbsp of melted coconut oil
Salt, pepper, turmeric, cayenne pepper and chili powder to taste

Method
Drain and wash all canned beans, place on kitchen paper to dry for 30 minutes, Preheat oven to 150 degrees fan assisted. Line a large baking tray with some baking parchment. Place beans and seeds in a large bowl, pour over melted coconut oil and sprinkle with seasoning and spices, mix until seeds and beans are coated well with oil and spices. Transfer onto lined baking tray and place in oven for around 2 hours or until beans have dried out. Remove from oven and allow to cool fully before enjoying a handful as a healthy snack.

Persian Inspired Aubergine and Walnut Dip
(Serves four)

Ingredients
2 large aubergines sliced in half
2 onions finely sliced
8 peeled garlic cloves
250g walnut halves
1tsp Himalayan pink salt
1tsp turmeric
1tbsp coconut palm sugar
2tbsp olive oil and a little extra to drizzle

Method
Preheat oven to 180 degrees fan assisted and line a baking tray with some foil. Place the garlic gloves and aubergine halves on the foil and sprinkle with the salt, turmeric and 1tbsp of the olive oil. Cover with foil and roast for around 40 minutes until aubergines are soft and cooked. While the aubergine is roasting, place the slices of onions, the remaining 1tbsp olive oil and coconut palm sugar into a large frying pan and fry on a low heat until the onions are cooked. In a food processor whiz up the walnuts to create a fine flour/ grain like consistency, take out a spoonful of the ground walnuts and set aside for later. Add the fried onions and mix on high speed until combined. Finally, when the aubergines are cooked, scoop out the flesh using a spoon and add to the food processor along with the roasted garlic cloves, mix for a good 5 minutes until well combined. Place into a serving dish, drizzle over a little olive oil and decorate with the ground walnuts. Delicious served with any raw vegetable.

Deserts
Who doesn't love a good desert? Although I don't think it's necessary to have desert every day, we should be able to enjoy the odd desert here and there and these recipes are not only delicious but healthy too!

Squidgy Chocolate Tray Bake
(Makes 16 squares)

Ingredients
150g stoned prunes
150g cooked butternut squash
80g cocoa powder
4 eggs
1 tin coconut milk
250g gluten free flour
1tsp baking powder
40g chia seeds
4tbs honey or pure maple syrup
100g organic butter or coconut oil if dairy free
Dried Rose petals to decorate (optional but looks pretty)
Method
Pre heat oven to 150 fan assisted. Place cocoa powder, flour, baking powder and chia seeds in a large mixing bowl. In a food processor whiz the coconut milk, butternut squash, eggs and prunes together, add to all dry ingredients and combine. Melt the butter and honey or maple syrup together over a low heat and pour into mixture, mix using a spatula until well combined. Pour the mixture into a lined brownie tray or a large lasagne dish and bake for 50 minutes. Allow to cool fully in the tray before sprinkling on the rose petals and cutting into squares.

Healthier Baklava
(Makes 24 squares)

This recipe has all the flavour and taste of traditional baklava but the texture is different as there is no pastry!

Ingredients
200g ground almonds
100g gluten free oats
2tbs chia seeds
200g nuts either pistachio or walnuts work well
100g melted coconut oil
100ml fresh coconut milk (not tinned)
1 tsp ground cardamom
1tsp ground cinnamon
1 cup of honey
½ tsp saffron
Zest of 1/2 orange
2tbsp rose water

Method
Place the ground almonds, oats, and chia seeds in a mixing bowl. Pour over the melted coconut oil and mix well. Pour in the fresh coconut milk and combine. Cover and leave to stand for 10 minutes. Pre heat oven to 150 fan assisted. Line a brownie tin with baking paper, place half of the mixture onto the baking paper and smooth down with the back of a metal spoon, when the tray has been covered evenly sprinkle 150g of the nuts and the ground cardamom and cinnamon over the mixture. Gently pat the remaining mixture over the nuts and pat down with back of metal spoon. Place into oven and bake for 25 minutes. Remove from oven and sprinkle on the remaining 50g nuts, allow to cool in tin and leave to 'set' for 3 hours. After 3 hours cut into diamond shapes but still leave in tin, in a small saucepan heat the honey, saffron water, orange zest and rose water until just reaches boiling point, do not allow to bubble away as the delicate flavours will be compromised. Gently Pour the hot honey mixture all over the baklava and be sure to pour in the groves where cut. Allow to cool and then place in fridge overnight, enjoy the following day.

Cashew and Date Fridge Bars
(Makes 16 bars)

Ingredients
300g pitted dates, soaked in water for 1 hour
275g raw cashew nuts
25g sesame seeds
1tsp vanilla extract
Method
Drain the dates and rinse under water, place into a high-speed blender and blend until smooth, add cashews and vanilla and blend on high speed until cashews are chopped to grain size pieces. Place mixture into a lined baking tray, sprinkle with sesame seeds and place in fridge overnight before cutting into bars.

Carrot and Walnut Cake with Creamy Frosting
(Serves 12)

Ingredients for the creamy frosting
200g cup raw cashews, soaked in water 2-3 hours and rinsed
2tbsp melted coconut oil
3tbsp honey
1 vanilla pod scraped
2 to 4tbsp of coconut milk water for blending

Ingredients for cake
300g grated carrot
4 eggs
250g honey
100g coconut palm sugar
200ml canned coconut milk
300ml pure sunflower oil
300g wholemeal spelt flour
1tsp baking powder
1tsp bicarbonate of soda
1 tsp Himalayan pink salt
2 tsp ground cinnamon
150g chopped walnuts

Method
Blend all frosting ingredients together in a high-speed blender until smooth and creamy, place in fridge for a few hours to thicken.

Pre-heat oven to 150 degrees fan assisted, line a baking tray with some baking parchment. In a food processor or cake mixer, mix together the eggs, honey, coconut palm sugar, coconut milk and sunflower oil, beat on high spend until mixed well. In a large bowl, sift together the spelt flour, baking powder, bicarbonate of soda, cinnamon and salt and add to the wet ingredients, mix on a slow speed until well incorporated, add the carrots and walnuts and using a spatula mix by hand for a couple of minutes. Pour the mixture into the lined baking tray, place in oven and cook for approximately 40 minutes; use a skewer to check cake is fully cooked before removing from oven, leave cake to cool in tin for 10 minutes before transferring onto a cooling rack to cool completely. Cover cake in frosting and decorate with walnuts

Dark Chocolate, Rum and Chestnut Brownies
(Makes 16 squares)

Ingredients
100g pitted dates
2tbsp boiling water
25ml dark rum
240g chestnut puree
4tbsp flax seeds
50g ground almonds
75g coconut flour
3 large organic eggs
150g organic butter
200g good quality dark chocolate (at least 85% cocoa)
200g coconut palm sugar

Method
Preheat oven to 160 degrees fan assist, line an 8" square baking tin with some baking parchment. Put the dates in a shallow bowl and pour the rum and 2tbsp boiling water over them, put aside and allow to soak for 30 minutes. After 30 minutes whizz the dates, and any remaining water/rum left over in the bowl through the food processor until you have a paste. In a separate mixing bowl separate the yolks and whites from the three eggs, put the whites aside for now and mix the yolks, chestnut puree, ground almonds, coconut palm sugar, flax seeds and coconut flour with a spatula until combined. Over a low heat melt the butter and chocolate together, pour into the above mixture and combine. Place the whites into a mixing bowl and beat on high until you have soft peaks, now gently fold the egg whites through the mixture, be careful not to mix too fast. Pour mixture into lined brownie tin and bake for 40 minutes Allow to cool in tin fully before turning out onto a plate to cut into squares. Tastes even better the next day!

Pear and Pistachio Loaf

(Makes 12 slices)

This loaf tastes even better the next day sliced and spread with almond or cashew butter....yum!

Ingredients
4 medium organic eggs
4 mashed bananas
4tbsp agave syrup
150ml melted coconut oil
200g rye flour
1tsp baking powder
1tsp bicarbonate of soda
4tbsp linseeds
100g dried pears, soaked for 30 minutes, drained and chopped 60g shelled and chopped pistachios (not salted or roasted)

Method

Preheat oven to 150 degrees fan assisted, line a 2lb loaf tin with some baking parchment. In a food processor or using an electric whisk, whisk the eggs for a few minutes then add the bananas, agave syrup and melted coconut oil, whizz on a high speed in the mixer for around 4 minutes. In a large bowl sift the rye flour, baking powder and bicarbonate of soda and add to the wet ingredients in the mixer. Use a medium speed to combine the ingredients in the mixer for a further 3 to 4 minutes until mixed well. Finally add the linseeds, pears and pistachio to the mixture and use a spatula to mix well by hand. Pour the mixture into the lined loaf tin and place in the oven. Bake for around 50 minutes. Remove from oven and use a skewer to test that the loaf has cooked all the way through by placing the skewer in the centre of the loaf, if it comes out clean it's cooked, if there is wet mixture on the skewer it needs to go back in the oven, check it every 10 minutes until cooked. Allow to cool in the loaf tin before slicing and serving.

Peanut Butter Cookies
(Makes 12)

These cookies are so yummy eaten warm fresh out the oven.
They will last around 1 to 2 days in an airtight container.

Ingredients
125g chickpea flour (also known as gram flour)
75g ground almonds
½ tsp bicarbonate of soda
1tbsp pure maple syrup
150g no added sugar peanut butter
Pinch of sea salt
150g coconut palm sugar
1 egg
Method
Mix all ingredients together and knead for a few minutes,
place in a large bowl and cover with cling film. Place bowl in
fridge for 2 hours. Pre heat oven to 160 degrees fan assisted
and line a baking sheet with some baking parchment. Remove
the cookie dough from the bowl and break into equal sized
portions approximately the size of a ping-pong ball, roll into a
ball shape and place on the baking sheet, gently press down
on each cookie dough ball to flatten slightly. Bake for around
10/ 12 minutes, being careful not to burn the cookies.

Blackberry, Coconut and Chocolate Torte
(Serves 12)

This torte is so rich and chocolaty it's sure to beat that chocolate craving!

Ingredients
50g raw cacao powder
200g melted coconut oil
100g of good quality dark chocolate (at least 85% cocoa solids)
4 large organic eggs
100g ground almonds
50g coconut flour
200g coconut palm sugar
50g dried coconut shavings
300g fresh blackberries

Method
Preheat oven to 150 degrees fan assisted and line an 8 inch round cake tin with some baking parchment. In a saucepan, on a low heat melt together the coconut oil and 100g of dark chocolate until smooth and set aside. Using a cake mixer or food processor, whisk the eggs and coconut palm sugar for 5 minutes before pouring into a large mixing bowl. Gently add the melted coconut oil and chocolate to the eggs, mix by hand using a spatula until combined. Sift the coconut flour, ground almonds and raw cacao powder into a separate bowl. Add to the wet ingredients by gently folding and mixing the flours until mixed well, finally add 200g of the blackberries to the mixture and gently mix. Pour the mixture into the lined cake tin and bake for 25-30 minutes or until a light crust forms on top and the torte is cooked (use the skewer method to check). Remove from the oven and allow to cool completely before removing from the tin. In a small sauce pan, place the remaining 100g blackberries in the pan and gently warm through for a few minutes until a little juice starts to release from the fruits, remove from the heat. Place the cooked and cooled torte on your cake stand or plate and pour the blackberries and their juice over the torte, finally decorate with the coconut shavings.

Thank You

Here comes the slushy, lovely bit where I want to thank all the people that have supported me throughout my journey.

To my husband and three beautiful children, I really cannot find the words to express how grateful I am for your continued support as you watched me go from an unhappy self-loathing woman to finding my own happiness with you all by my side. You loved me when I didn't love myself and gave me the strength to reach my weight loss goals and have provided me with endless support as I've worked hard to maintain my day job, writing this book and trying to be the best Mum and wife that I can. I love you all from the bottom of my heart.

To my parents who very kindly paid for me to have weight loss surgery knowing that it was my last resort, my last attempt at happiness. You cannot imagine how grateful I am for everything you have done to give me a new start in life, from funding my surgery through to looking after your grandchildren whilst I work and your encouragement as I wrote this book.

To my friends and family... Too many of you to name individually, but rest assured that every single one of you who stood by me as I found my way to becoming who I am today has played a huge part in my journey. From the friends who know me so well that I can cry with and tell them everything to the friends that I've met through social media and who have supported me as I reached my target. You are all special to me and have inspired me no end to write this book.

Last but not least, thank YOU for reading this book and I hope it brings you much success in your own journey.

The most precious word in the dictionary ... Thank You!

Truly Nourished
Health & Lifestyle Coaching

Hali offers personal one to one coaching in Bristol and surrounding areas.

To find out more about Health and Lifestyle Coaching with Hali Jafari, take a look at the Truly Nourished website

www.trulynourished.co.uk

A special thank you to Karen Lowe for use of her gorgeous kitchen during the photo shoot and help with styling. You can find out more about Karen's work by visiting her website.
www.karenl.co.uk

Photography credit Viktoria Kuti a talented photographer based in Bristol please find her at:
www.viktoriakuti.com

Cover design by creative designer Ellie Bowie, please check out her work:
www.eleanorbowie.co.uk

Notes…

Notes…

Notes…

Printed in Great Britain
by Amazon